Tonsil Stones

The Truth about Tonsil Stones

(Eliminate Tonsil Stones and Have Fresh Breath in Just Days!)

Joshua Levine

Published By **Darby Connor**

Joshua Levine

All Rights Reserved

Tonsil Stones: The Truth about Tonsil Stones (Eliminate Tonsil Stones and Have Fresh Breath in Just Days!)

ISBN   978-1-990373-95-4

No part of this guidebook shall be reproduced in any form without permission in writing from the publisher except in the case of brief quotations embodied in critical articles or reviews.

Legal & Disclaimer

The information contained in this book is not designed to replace or take the place of any form of medicine or professional medical advice. The information in this book has been provided for educational & entertainment purposes only.

The information contained in this book has been compiled from sources deemed reliable, and it is accurate to the best of the Author's knowledge; however, the Author cannot guarantee its accuracy and validity and cannot be held liable for any errors or omissions. Changes are periodically made to this book. You must consult your doctor or get professional medical advice before using any of the suggested remedies, techniques, or information in this book.

Table Of Contents

Chapter 1: The Tonsils Revealed

First and foremost, it is important and necessary to understand the anatomy of the throat and what tonsils exactly are before we explore the nature and treatments of tonsil stones. After all, if we can better understand the organ in its normal, healthy state, we may be better prepared to protect ourselves against unhealthily behavior and its consequences.

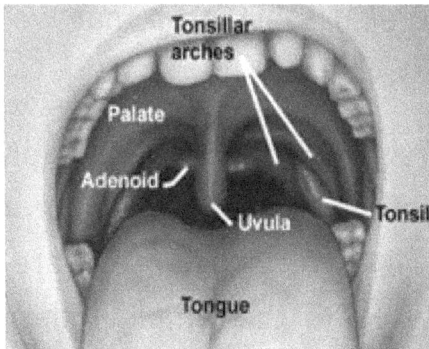

As we can see by the diagram below there are actually three pairs of tonsils in the throat. The pharyngeal tonsils (a.k.a.

the adenoids) are located behind your nose. The two palatine tonsils are located on both sides of the back of the throat (also what most people refer to when they talk about tonsils). Finally, the lingual tonsils are located at the back of the tongue (not pictured).

Alright, so we now know the names and locations of our tonsils, but what is it that they exactly do? Well, they are part of the lymphatic system and their primary function is to provide a barrier from foreign substances that we inhale or ingest.

The foreign substances we are primarily talking about her are bacteria or viruses. These foreign substances are then transported to the lymph nodes where they are taken out into a back alley and roughed up and told that they need to leave town pronto.

However, when your tonsils become infected or otherwise compromised, it can leave you susceptible to a whole host of problems. Obviously, this is where tonsil stones come in. That is, if your tonsils are struggling to function or are functioning poorly due to tonsil stones then in effect your whole body is susceptible to infection and disease.

So how does one exactly get tonsil stones? And if one does get tonsil stones, how would one go about treating them? Also, is there any way to avoid getting tonsil stones in the first place? These are all excellent questions and are exactly what we plan to discuss in this e-Book.

The Mystery of the Stones

Before we get into what exactly tonsil stones are, it may be helpful to understand that tonsils are not an integral part of the body. At least, they are not anymore. It is believed that tonsils used to play a larger role in the defense against bacteria and disease. However, current studies show that those who have had part or all of their tonsils removed are no more likely to develop colds and flu viruses or other pathogens than are those who have all of their tonsils.

This is all to say that you should remember to keep an ounce of reason in your mix of tonsil stone understanding. That is, there is no reason to feel like it is a symptom of a larger illness or that somehow the pain in your throat is an indication of further future swelling that will eventually shut of your air pipe. These ideas are unfounded.

That said, if you are like many people, you have not heard of tonsil stones (a.k.a. tonsilloliths). If you haven't heard of tonsil stones do not feel like you have not been paying attention to the latest in medical discoveries, as it is not a fatal condition.

However, because it will not kill you while driving your kids to school doesn't mean that it shouldn't be given the proper attention. Later on this eBook we will discuss some of the consequences of tonsil stones and how you can mitigate the severity of them, but for now understand those that suffer from tonsil stones do indeed have a serious medical condition.

Simply put, tonsil stones are the result of collections of calcified material forming in your tonsils. For the most part, these formations do not occur in the adenoids, but rather they form primarily in the palatine tonsils and sometimes the lingual.

The actual process of developing tonsil stones is not too complicated. Imagine if you will your tonsils as having a bunch of little nooks and crevices. Now imagine that these little nooks and crevices have some debris caught within them. This debris begins to calcify over time and next thing you know you have tonsilloliths.

Basically the debris caught in your tonsils is the same as a grain of sand in an oyster; the difference is your tonsils aren't going to produce expensive pearls!

It has been documented most people who develop these stones also have frequent tonsil infections. Now, these tonsil infections can be in any of the three pairs of tonsils, but as stated before, the actual development of tonsil stones typically occurs in the palatine or lingual tonsils.

What is also important to know about this condition is it also comes in a variety of forms. That is, many people have these stones but they do not know it because they have not caused significant discomfort.

If you know you have these stones and do not experience an adverse effects then you can consider yourself lucky, but you also need to realize that these stones can continue to grow if you do nothing about them. This is again to say that an ounce of prevention is worth a pound of cure.

Some of the symptoms and discomfort that may be indicators of tonsil stones include:

Feeling as if you need to clear your throat constantly

Itching or tickling feeling in the throat

Pain when swallowing

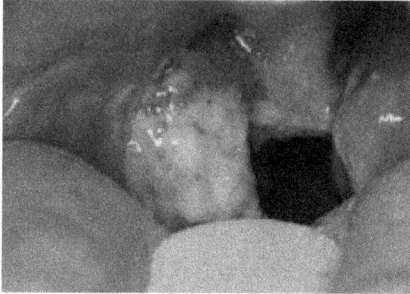

Tenderness in the throat when eating

Swollen areas in the back of the throat

Redness and irritation of the tonsils

White debris on and around the tonsils

Bad breath

All of these symptoms are indicative of tonsil stones, or at the very least a buildup of bacteria in the throat and tonsil area.

The Cause (and Bane) of Stones

Hopefully, by this point, you've gained an appreciation for what these stones truly are. If not, let's do a quick recap.

Tonsil stones are the result of debris that has caught in the nooks and crevices of your tonsils and begun to calcify. These calcifications, while uncomfortable and often embarrassing because they cause halitosis, are not life threatening and can be managed through a number of effective techniques.

Myths

The reason it's important to reiterate what these stones are is so we can keep our minds in a scientific mind frame. If you've ever gone online and tried to do some research on the condition, you know that there are a number of sites out there that seem more interested in being interesting than being factual.

It is not worth giving credence to these myths by expanding on them here, but know that there are really only three widely accepted ways that these stones come about. They are listed below.

Causes

The first cause is natural, that it is often a result of nature just being nature. For example, sometimes mucous or dead cells become trapped in these nooks and crevices and then begin to harden.

What this means is that many times those who have these stones are not directly responsible for them. Not that any of us would judge an individual with a medical issue, but there are sometimes myths exchanged amongst people that tonsil stones are a result of unhealthy living. While a lack of oral care is also a cause of these stones, it doesn't mean the individual is a bad person.

With proper oral care, however, a person can reduce the chances of them developing this condition. The reasoning is simple: the more you take care of your mouth, the less likely debris has a chance to linger and develop into something worse.

A final cause is related to tonsillitis. More specifically, it has been scientifically demonstrated that those who sufferer repeated bouts of tonsillitis are also more susceptible to contracting these stones.

The relations between the two is currently being studied, but the common sense approach tells us because of the constant instability with this particular organ, that it allows itself to trap particle so debris and bacteria more easily and thus provide the nascent building blocks of tonsil stones.

Again though, it bears repeating that tonsil stones are not due to a person who is living an immoral lifestyle or who are purposely neglectful. These stones are more than likely a result of living in an imperfect world.

Chapter 2: How Do You Know If You Have Them?

If there is anything good about this condition it is there are numerous signs and symptoms. What this means is that for most of us, we will be able to tell very easily if we need to go to the doctor.

Below is list of many of the indicators that something is wrong with your tonsils but remember that it is not comprehensive list. That is, some symptoms may arise that are not listed here. The point being is that if you suspect there is issues seek medical attention as soon as possible.

White Debris

This can easily be confirmed by a simple visual inspection. If you check your tonsils and notice that there is a white growth occurring than you have stones. Remember though some people have stones that are small enough not to be seen, so just because you don't see white debris but have other symptoms doesn't mean you are stone free.

Pain

This may be the most common symptom. Why? Well, the simple reason that your throat has been physically altered is a good reason. Your throat is used to functioning in a certain way, and when a relatively quick growth occurs the machinery in your throat tends to grind. The pain doesn't have to be debilitating but even if it is barely noticeable you may want to consider getting it check out.

Difficulty Swallowing

This may be the easiest self-examination procedure you can give yourself. That is, by simply taking a few gulps of some water you can determine if there are problems with your tonsils. Yes, it may seem like a crude and inaccurate test, but all you need do is put the tonsils to work to see if they respond positively or negatively to stress.

Inflammation

This is another simple visual check. Of course, not all of us know what our tonsils look like normally, but for the most part inflammation is detectable. When you see inflamed redness then it's time to take action. Again, if you suspect something is amiss though, please consult with your doctor.

Coughing

This is a great symptom in there is no subjectivity involved. Unlike the visual check of seeing if the tonsils are inflamed, coughing will absolutely tell you that something is wrong. Again, please remember coughing alone is obviously not enough to determine if you have stones. In conjunction with a number other symptoms, however, it should raise some red flags.

Sore Throat

This almost goes hand in hand with coughing, especially if you are coughing a lot. Be mindful of how your throat feels and you may discover a larger issue as to why.

Fatigue

This is mostly related to the growth's irritation of the throat, which results in coughing. You might not think it but coughing takes an inordinate amount of physical energy. In addition, when you cough consistently your brain may associate with sickness and thus make you feel fatigued.

Halitosis

What is that smell? Yes, it might be your breath; breath that can knock a sleeping cow over because it is so pungent. This pungency is primarily due to the stones that are growing in your mouth. Remember, these stones are calcified debris.

Pain in the Ear

Let's not forget we are holistic beings, meaning nothing happens in a vacuum. When our throats have something wrong with them it can often affect nearby organs and systems. It's because of this when we notice ear pain, it might be a result of something wrong with our throats.

What's important to remember is none of these symptoms on their own necessarily mean anything. It is only in combination with each they add up to a possible condition of tonsil stones. If you have any suspicions that you may have this condition, regardless of if you are presenting with these symptoms, it is imperative you seek medical attention as soon as possible.

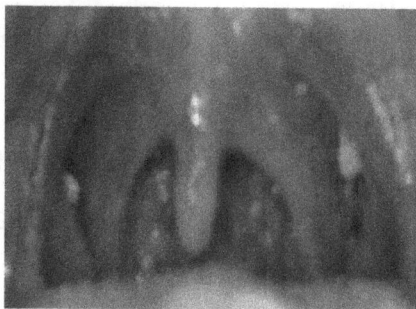

The Master Secret No One Will Ever Tell You About

For those of us who have gone through the pain of tonsil stones, we know we never want to have to go through it again. However, it is not like we have complete control over our bodies, none of us does, so is it even possible to control whether your body develops tonsil stones.

The short answer is no. Despite all the advancements made with science and the understanding of ourselves, we cannot control numerous aspect of how our body will respond to certain conditions. That's why symptoms to stones, though scary and at the very least annoying, can be considered a good thing. After all, it is beneficial to receive a little warning, which is all a symptom is, that our body is having a problem.

This all leads up to the question: How can we manage the possibility of our body developing stones? Well, the good news is you do have some control over that.

What's odd though is despite this information having the potential of helping millions of people, there are some strategies to developing a lifestyle that's conducive to not developing stones people won't tell you about. Why this is exactly, who's to say? The point is there's one great way to avoid stones you probably never heard of: avoid dairy.

Dairy Is a Not a Friend

We've been told since we were kids we need milk and dairy in our lives so we can develop strong bones and muscles. And there is no contesting the scientific evidence dairy can help with the development and maintenance of these body parts.

However, dairy also causes some specific reactions in the body that can cause a person to be much more likely to develop stones.

How this works is like this: when you drink milk or use dairy products your body has a tendency to produce more mucus. This excessive production is especially true if you are allergic to dairy products. This increased production can either drip down the back of your throat where it becomes caught in the crevices and nooks of your tonsils, or it can simply be not flushed out of your throat where it again finds its way into your tonsils.

As we've stated before, once this mucous sits in your tonsils where it may or may not trap more debris, it will begin to harden and calcify and then you have the beginning of a stone. By avoiding unnecessary dairy, you can reduce your chances of developing this condition.

Now, you may ask, how if dairy is a necessary part of an individual's diet then how can you completely cut dairy out. Well, the answer to that is you do not completely cut dairy out. What you do is begin to use dairy supplements. These supplements can come in any number of forms such as pills or powders, and can often be found in the supermarkets and grocery stores that you are buying your milk in the first place.

It also begs the question though; do you really know what a dairy product is? Of course we know milk and butter and cheese are, but what are some of the less commonly known dairy products? Below is a list of the most common:

Custard

Nougat

Margarine (not all brands, but many)

Pudding

Whey

Yogurt

So if all of these products are dairy products, what are some of the products you can replace these with? And remember, everything you enjoy now that contains dairy can still be enjoyed because food producers have created so many alternatives to satisfy those who have dairy allergies. This is to say that it is not like you'll have to undergo a major lifestyle change.

Again, below is a list of the most common substitutions:

Cocoa Butter

Creamed Tartar

Creamed Honey

Soymilk Powder

Vegan Cheese

Gluten-free Yogurt

Ultimately, this is all to say while you may not be able to completely control everything your body does or how it reacts, you can mitigate the chances of developing or worsening stones but reducing or replacing your dairy intake.

60-Day Prevention Plan to Keep Tonsil Stones at Bay

As stated several times in this eBook, tonsil stones do not have to be some kind of debilitating condition. In fact, research about this condition is sometimes slow to develop because it lacks the priority of cancer, diabetes, and all those other big name conditions.

However, know that it can become serious, but you don't let it have to. In fact, if you've discovered you have tonsil stones, you can keep them at bay and possibly even eliminate them within 60 days.

How? Well there are a number of ways, but this eBook concentrates on the most efficient ones.

Over the next four chapters you will have the best methods to manage or reduce your tonsil stones. So, without further adieu let's learn about:

Continuing with Good Oral Health Care

Focusing on a Healthy Diet

Maintaining an Alkaline Environment

Using a Liver Cleanse

Continuing with Good Oral Health

Good oral health care is considered a major foundation in the fight against tonsil stones. After all, tonsils are a result of an accumulation of debris being allowed to sit long enough to calcify and grow. By continuing with good oral care, you can remove this debris before it is allowed to accumulate. How? Below are a number of tried and true simple strategies to keeping your mouth (and subsequently your tonsils) clean.

Chapter 3: Brushing Your Teeth

Yes, we all know brushing our teeth is important. (Our mother's told us as much for most of our childhoods). Still, it is doubtful you brush as often or as effectively as you should.

The ADA recommends you brush your teeth at least twice a day and also strongly recommends you bush immediately after meals. They give this recommendation for the same reason brushing helps prevent tonsil stones. That is, by brushing away all of the debris that can cause tooth decay and gum problems, you are also brushing away all the debris that can cause tonsil stones. Here are a few basic reminders of how to brush your teeth.

1. You want to have the brush at about a 45 degree angle against the gum line, and then you want to sweep or roll the

brush away. Do not think of your teeth as a tile floor with a stain on it that you'll only get out by vigorously scrubbing. You want to remove the debris, not the enamel.

2. Don't forget there are three sides to your teeth: the top, the back, and the front. You need to get all three sides to make sure all debris is removed.

3. Finally, don't forget to brush your tongue. Your tongue (aside from your gums) is the biggest host of bacteria; bacteria that cannot only cause tonsil stones, but also just plain old bad breath.

Flossing Your Teeth

In addition to keeping your mouth clean through brushing, you should also floss. The ADA recommends at least once a day because, again, this is how you keep your mouth and throat in health working order. Here are a few reminders on flossing.

1. You should only need about a foot and half of floss for your entire mouth. Any less and you may be reusing floss that has debris on it and thus reinserting into your mouth.

2. Don't think of the floss as a band saw cutting through dense lumber. Your gums should not be bleeding profusely. Simply put, follow the gentle curves of your teeth.

3. Don't forget about under the gum line. Again, you don't need to dig in, but you will need to get as close to the bend of the tooth as possible.

Rinse, Please!

Finally, the last step in oral care that will reduce your stones in 60 days (or prevent them altogether) is by rinsing.

Unlike brushing and flossing, it's tough to develop bad habits with rinsing (the only one being not doing it), but remember you should keep the rinse in your mouth for about two minutes.

The flossing not only removes some of the physical debris, but more importantly it actively fights against the bacteria in your mouth. Our mouths have many pockets that flossing and brushing cannot get to frequently enough. Rinsing is often the only way to make sure that your entire mouth is immaculate.

However, make sure you are using a therapeutic mouth rinse and not a cosmetic one. Cosmetic ones only freshen breath. Below are some commonly used rinses ADA approved therapeutic mouth rinses.

ACT Anti-cavity Fluoride Rinse

Care One Antiseptic Mouth rinse

Crest Pro-Health

CVS Antiseptic Mouth Rinse

Equate Anti-cavity Fluoride Rinse

Rite Aid Antiseptic Mouth Rinse

Swan Spring Antiseptic Mouth Rinse

No matter what kind of rinse you use it is important to swish and gargle the rinse in your mouth for at least 2 minutes for maximum antibacterial and flushing action.

Diet

What isn't diet connected to? It seems as if every ailment or malady can be reduced or eliminated through an improved diet. Why? Because the facts are the food you put in your body have a significant effect on the way you think and feel. Your diet and its relationship to tonsil stones are no different.

The problem being is we are so poorly educated about our diets to begin with; there's is no way we would naturally know what foods may be complicit in the development of tonsil stones.

Below are some of the generally accepted foods you should avoid if you want to reduce or prevent tonsil stones.

Foods to Avoid

Mostly, you want to avoid foods that are inherently high in bacteria to begin with. This category would include most dairy products and many meat products. Obviously, if the food product is from another animal than it will be higher in bacteria. These foods would include but are not limited to:

Eggs

Steak

Ground Beef

Bacon

Ham

Poultry

However, you should also keep your digestive system in an alkaline environment. We'll get more into that in the next chapter, but the idea is you want to lessen the acidity in your system. The acid, as many of you well know, can be caustic and leave your tonsils more susceptible to infection. Food products to avoid would include:

Tomato based sauces

Coffee

Strong Tea

Liquor

Beer

Soda

Other Carbonated beverages

If you're looking for a low acid diet plan you can check out diet plans for people with stomach ulcers. The goal of reducing acid and providing soothing foods and drinks doesn't mean you have to give up everything you love to eat but you must learn moderation and the effect that the acidic foods and drinks may have on your health from your stomach and digestive tract to your tonsils.

Chapter 4: Helpful Foods

On the other side of that diet coin, there are foods that can actually help you thwart the growth of tonsil stones or actually prevent them. It is important to understand though, that these foods are not some magic cure. That is, you don't simply eat them once or twice a week and know that your tonsil stones will have magically disappeared.

It should be remembered with any attempt to improve your health, the change will not occur overnight. It is imperative as an individual that you make a commitment to this new lifestyle. This includes making sure you are incorporating the foods listed below into your daily diet.

Celery

The major benefit that celery brings is the production of saliva. That is, when we eat celery our mouths produce slightly more saliva. And as we all know saliva contains chemicals help break down food and kill bacteria. Simply put, the more saliva the less bacteria gets a chance to infect your tonsils.

Cucumber

Don't like this bland food? Well, oddly enough it can help you reduce tonsil stones through its properties. How's that? Because it is a fibrous food it helps remove some of the tartar and bacteria in your mouth. Thus, less bacteria and debris available to calcify in the nooks and crannies of your tonsils.

Apple

Apples are fiber rich fruits that help clean your teeth to remove tarter and debris from your mouth.

Onion

I know, when you think of onions you instantly think of bad breath, but wouldn't you rather have the odor of onions than of bacteria growing on your tonsils? Onions are a natural and powerful bacteria killing food. You can always chew some parsley or mint leaves afterwards to freshen your breath.

Wasabi

With Wasabi, you get two great benefits for the price of one. Not only can you spice up your Japanese food (or hot dog if you're into that kind of thing), but because of the properties of this condiment, you can also destroy a vast number of bacteria in your mouth. Destroying bacteria before it has a chance to migrate to your tonsils is always a benefit, careful though, this stuff is strong!

Shitake Mushroom

Do you see a pattern in the foods that are recommended to reduce or prevent tonsil stones? If so, that's good because this one is no different. A Shitake mushroom, which just so happens to be delicious to begin with, is also a great source of anti-bacterial food. Again, incorporate throughout your diet. You can't just eat one of these guys a week and expect to be OK.

H20

Even though this obviously isn't a food, it is a liquid that is very important in the maintenance of your mouth's health. We all need water to stay hydrated anyway, and by doing so you also improve your immune system, but the simple act of drinking water removes most of the loose debris in your mouth.

It is like mouth rinse except without all the fancy chemicals to kill bacteria.

Gargling with plain old water can help flush the nooks and crannies of your tonsils to move debris on down the throat to be eliminated from the body.

Take every opportunity to include these items in your diet, add them to salads, have an apple for dessert or include them in soups and meals as much as possible.

An Alkaline Environment is the Key to Rapid Success

Many of you may have heard about alkaline diets. There's a reason for this, as alkaline diets have shown themselves to have numerous healthy benefits. However, what exactly is an alkaline diet? You may think creating an alkaline environment means eliminating acidic foods, in fact the designation of a food as alkaline or acid refers to the residue left once the foods have been digested.

So, citrus fruits which are often considered to be acidic actually are alkaline producers within the digestive tract

An alkaline diet typically consists of whole foods, especially fruits, vegetables, and root crops. This diet also includes nuts, seeds, spices, whole grains, and beans. Alkalizing beverages, like spring water and green tea, are also essential elements of this diet.

The key to an alkaline environment is to avoid processed and artificial foods, caffeine, white sugar, and white flour when possible. However, you can use real butter and full-cream milk. For cooking and lending to your alkaline diet you should only use virgin olive oil, coconut oil, and avocado oil.

This can seem to be a very limited diet considering the typical American diet includes meat, dairy, saturated fats, sugar, alcohol and caffeine. These items can cause a buildup of acid wastes in the body that are a perfect environment ground for yeasts, fungus, molds, bacteria, and viruses and must be significantly limited in daily use.

Because alkaline diet excludes families of foods including meat, poultry, cheese and grains it can lead to a diet that is off balance and deficient in many fatty acids, protein and calcium. While you can work to achieve an alkaline environment in your body it is not advised that you do this long term. Achieving a healthy balance between acids and alkalinity is the goal.

However there are things you can do to promote a healthy balance and reduction of acid in your body thus helping create a hostile environment for bacteria and debris that would form tonsil stones.

Besides your oral health the overall health of your body and the digestive tract plays a huge part in your susceptibility to bacteria and tonsil stones. Eating a healthy diet, practicing good oral health habits and your knowledge about tonsil stones are a good start, but to help create a healthy environment in your body you may want to also do a liver cleanse.

The Liver Cleanse Rids Toxins and Keeps Stones Away

This liver cleanse is a traditional home remedy that has been passed down among naturopaths and home remedy fans for generations. The natural process of flushing your liver and cleansing it for maximum efficiency and health can affect all the other aspects of your bodily health.

The liver is responsible for removing fat soluble toxins and other waste from your body. It is best to do a liver cleanse when you don't have a lot of things going on and don't need to work. Typically you are looking at three days of flushing during which you will carefully decide what to ingest.

A simple liver cleanse program:

For two days drink two glasses of organic apple juice every two hours.

During the first 24 hours eat nothing.

On the second day eat only fresh fruits and vegetables.

At bedtime on the second day mix two tablespoons of Epsom salts in a glass of water.

Drink the water and then drink half a cup of olive oil mixed with two teaspoons of lemon juice.

Olive oil and the Epsom salts will cause you to feel nauseous and you may not get much sleep, but try to remain prone and rest as much as possible. If you need to go to the bathroom do so.

When you wake up in the morning you may have some cramping then you'll feel a pressure building in your intestines. Go to the bathroom to void your bladder and bowels and voila! You've cleansed your liver.

The reason that this plan works to cleanse your liver is the science involved and how the things you eat and drink work inside your body.

Apple juice contains a large amount of malic acid that works to weaken adhesions holding solid fatty deposits together in your body. Vegetables and fruits provide fiber. Epsom salts relax and dilate the bile duct allowing the waste to pass through completely. Pure olive oil stimulates the bile duct to expel waste.

Again, a liver cleanse is a beneficial treatment that will help regulate many of the different cycles of the body and improve your overall health.

Safely Removing Tonsil Stones Yourself

Okay, typically it is not recommended you attempt medical procedures at home but you can safely remove tonsil stones yourself. There are two methods which you can use.

Method One for Removing Tonsil Stones at Home

What you'll need to remove your tonsil stones are basically common household and medicine cabinet items.

Cotton swabs

Mirror

Oxygenating Mouthwash

Flashlight

Once you've gathered all your supplies it's time to get started. You may want to have a family member assist you because there are a lot of things to juggle all at once.

Moisten the cotton swab 'til it is damp but not dripping.

Hold a mirror and flashlight in front of your face with the same hand or in your assistant's hand so that you can open your mouth and have full visibility of the back of your throat.

Use the cotton swab to sweep each tonsil dislodging debris and tonsil stones. You can also poke on the outer fold of the tonsils to express hidden stones. Take care not to push the stones further into the folds and nooks of the tonsil.

After you've carefully removed all the stones and debris from your tonsils gargle and rinse well with an oxygenating mouthwash.

Method Two for Removing Tonsil Stones at Home

The second method requires the same instruments except instead of a cotton swab you'll be using an oral irrigator. Some people use both of these methods to ensure that they've truly removed all the stones and debris from their tonsils.

Following the same steps as in method one to view and access your tonsils use an oral irrigator on the lowest setting to irrigate and flush your tonsils. Avoid any higher settings which could cause your tonsils to become irritated, bleed and possibly get infected.

Once you've flushed the tonsils and removed all the stones and debris gargle and rinse well with an oxygenating mouthwash.

Removing tonsil stones at home is not difficult and as long as you are careful not to irritate or damage the tonsils there is no reason why you should not do this yourself. If you don't see any evidence of tonsil stones but are experiencing many of the symptoms you may have infected tonsils or tonsillitis. If that is the case it is important that you seek a professional treatment.

Chapter 5: Alternative Methods In Removing Tonsil Stones

Besides the methods described previously there are other ways to go about removing and indeed preventing tonsil stones. Over the years there have been many home remedies for sore throats, painful swallowing etc. Many people did not realize that they likely were suffering from tonsil stones. These home remedies are natural and will not harm your body, as well as providing relief from tonsil stones and their symptoms.

Gargling

Gargling provides flushing of the tonsils as well as helping relive pain and irritation along with improving halitosis. There are several gargle ingredients that provide relief, just a few include:

Hot salt water gargle helps with swelling and pain in the throat and tonsils as well as flushing the tonsils to remove debris.

Alum salt mixed with warm water makes a great tonsil gargle.

Mint mouthwash can flush the tonsils and help eliminated bad breath as well as helping prevent formation of tonsil stones.

Colloidal silver gargle provides relief from pain and irritation as well as removing tonsil stones.

Home Remedies and Herbals

Swallow a spoonful of turmeric powder and sugar followed by sipping hot water to reduce tonsil stones.

Mix one pinch of finely powdered mustard with water and gargle to relieve irritation.

Mix one quarter teaspoon of salt, four teaspoons of honey and the juice of a fresh lemon into a glass of water for a tasty lemonade drink that you can sip to relieve tonsil irritation and pain.

Make a hot tea with sweet violet flowers and water. Boil, steep and filter then drink hot to relieve irritation and inflammation in the tonsils.

Simmer two tablespoons of fenugreek seeds for half an hour in one liter of water. Allow to cool and use as a soothing gargle to reduce inflammation and flush the tonsils.

When Natural Methods Fail it's Time for a Doctor's Help

If you have a severe case or a recurring problem with tonsil stones you may wish to consider medical treatments. While many people prefer to avoid the extreme measures which most medical procedures involve for anything involving the tonsils or throat, there are several options to choose from.

Curettage

Curettage is, to put it simply, a surgical procedure where the stone is removed with a curette. Sure it sounds quick and easy but this is a surgery and you will face all the usual risks involved with surgery. Anesthesia, infection, pain etc.

Resurfacing

Resurfacing the tonsils involves a laser being used to vaporize the surface of the tonsils, thus removing the nooks and crannies leaving no place for the stones to form.

Tonsil Removal

A tonsillectomy is the most drastic response to tonsil stones, and involves the complete removal of the tonsils.

Each of these procedures is invasive, can be painful and places you at the risk of infection. They also may require you to miss work in order to recover.

In the case of curettage you could go through all that pain and then still grow new tonsil stones, if you don't make the changes in your diet, oral health and lifestyle to prevent them from forming.

Even with a full tonsillectomy or resurfacing the bacteria that causes the odor and irritation in your tonsils will still be present, only it may now attach to other areas of your throat which can cause more problems.

Tonsil Stones Banished Forever!

The annoyance, odor and yes, even pain of tonsil stones can disrupt your life, damage your eating habits and make you feel bad as well. You may not think that something as small as a tonsil stone could affect your overall health.

But when you consider that they are formed from bacteria it's easy to imagine how having a bacterial laden area in your throat could lead to stomach problems, digestive infections and even heartburn and indigestion as well as lethargy and weakness. You are essentially breeding infection in your throat!

Start today to improve your oral hygiene habits, eradicate existing tonsil stones and adjust your diet and lifestyle to prevent future occurrences!

There's no need to go through invasive surgeries, painful procedures and long recovery periods. You now have the information and the tools you need to eliminate tonsil stones from your life without a visit to the doctor.

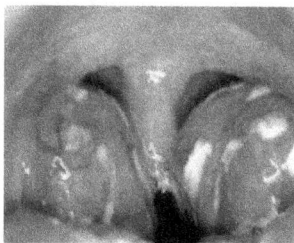

Tonsil stones may be annoying and even painful, but there are many ways to alleviate the symptoms and relieve your tonsils of this debris and buildup! You don't have to live with the irritation, bad

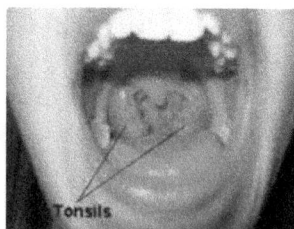

breath and scratchy throat associated with tonsil stones.

Take your tonsils from this:

To this:

In just 60 short days you can rid yourself
of tonsil stones and restore your mouth,
tonsils and throat to a healthy germ-free
environment!

Chapter 6: Caseum And Candidiasis, What Is The Report?

One of the main reason for having white ball-like structures within the throat can be candidiasis. It's a kind of yeast infection that can affect various areas in the oral cavity in the way we understand it.

It affects the top part of the tongue. But it may extend to the throat. This causes the formation of white ball within the throat. The type of infection caused by yeast is extremely uncommon, but it's important to note that the spreading of throat infections is usually seen when people have poor immune systems.

Salt water. Studies have shown that rinsing with salt water can be a very effective remedy of mouth sores.

Yogurt. Yogurt containing probiotics could reduce the amount of bacteria that cause tonsil stone.

Apples. Their acid content aids in fighting bacteria within the tonsils.

Carrots. Chewing carrots increases saliva production and naturally occurring antibacterial substances. This may help to lessen or even eliminate the need for tonsil calculs.

Onions. They are thought to have powerful antibacterial qualities. Incorporating them into your diet may help to prevent or remove tonsillar stones.

Lasers are used to treat

If treatment and cleaning is not enough to resolve the issue, you can try another method. In reality, according to the degree of discomfort that is felt by the patient ENT may opt to use laser. The physician will pass the laser over the tonsils for five to ten seconds at a time in various places.

The laser creates areas of impact, and then vaporizes tonsils. They're burned onto the surface. They then decrease in their size when the laser passes. At the end of the day, they appear black and are thinner and are well-hidden within their cavity.

The 10 minutes of treatment are uncomfortable for the patient, even with an anesthetic spray however, the procedure is somewhat uncomfortable. After three sessions in average there's a noticeable reduction in the secretions of the caseum.

Make sure to rinse your mouth after every meal.

As we eat, food particles get stored within the mouth nooks and crannies in the mouth. Don't forget to wash your mouth every meal with the best oxygenated brand of mouthwash.

Remove Regular Stones

It is possible to help remove tonsils of stones every day with an swab of cotton. Utilizing a cotton swab, or your finger to apply pressure along the bottom of the stones. Continue to apply the pressure. If it gets soft, slide it over the stone until you can gently take it off the stone. After that, rinse your mouth with mouthwash.

Dental Irrigation Syringes : These irrigation syringes have an ergonomically shaped plastic tip could be used to distribute mouthwash, or to wash the caseum. Then, you can direct the syringe's point at the pockets of your tonsils to wash the pockets.

Much more effective than the cotton swabs, it helps to dislodge stones that are inserted deep within the tonsils. Maintain your head in a neutral position while performing this process to stop tonsil stones from falling into the lining of your throat.

The Irrigator: It is possible to purchase a water jet it is a jet for dental use fitted with a tank of water to eliminate all debris from the mouth cavity. This allows for perfect dental hygiene, and it is highly recommended by dentists.

The spray was developed to replace dental floss, but it could also be used to get rid of tonsil casesum. But, you must be cautious not to use too much force using the spray for your tonsils so as to prevent damaging them. Make sure you apply it on the side of the tonsil's pocket, in which the caseum can be found.

Another option is to eliminate the inequalities. Radiofrequency and Cauterization performed with local anesthesia may cause burning of the inequalities on the surface. Additionally, you can remove them using freezing (cryotherapy).

To avoid having to undergo this procedure, the most effective option is to utilize the CO_2 laser. The operation is carried out at any time during the day under local anesthesia. The patient is discharged from the hospital 2 hours after the procedure. A minimum of two to four sessions are needed, depending on the intensity of the laser as well as the state of the tonsils.

At the end of the day, they experienced a form that is known as "peeling" but they continue to perform their job in the field of infection prevention. Very well done.

This method can result in a treatment in between 80 and 90 percentage of instances.

Chapter 7: What Are The Main Risk Factors?

Similar to all ailments there are a variety of factors that can trigger tonsillitis.

Smoking cigarettes or being exposed to smoke from secondhand sources

Go to "at risk" places: Daycares, schools, hospitals, and so on.

You should be alert to the presence of chemicals that cause irritation (household chemicals, pesticides etc.)

Being afflicted with a low immune system as a result of other illnesses (HIV or cancer, diabetes, etc.)

Chronic infections that affect the respiratory system, such as sinusitis, bronchitis and so on.

Tonsillitis is a common cause of infection.

Tonsillitis originating from bacteria The most prevalent, is very infectious. It can be transmitted by in direct or in indirect contact (projection of infectious droplets) in the respiratory secretions of someone who is carrying.

If not treated with antibiotics, tonsillitis caused streptococci could remain infected for three weeks after onset symptoms. But, the research suggests that the possibility of contracting decreases to a minimum after just 24 hours of treatment.

Home Remedies to get rid of casesum made with sea salt

Salt is a healthy component that has antiseptic as well as antibacterial properties. It will aid in the elimination of white balls in the throat keep your throat clear and well-maintained.

Chapter 8: How Do You Remove The Salt Caseum From Your Body?

Ingredients

One teaspoon sea salt

The glass is filled with water.

Measures

Place some water into the microwave or in a pan.

If it's boiling Remove from the flame and sprinkle sea salt on top.

Take the liquid out with an ice cube so that salt disintegrates more easily.

Are you ready to try this natural gargle at the end of every meal.

So you can remove caseum through a straightforward procedure because saltwater will create these ball-like structures from tonsils that you are able to eliminate effortlessly. Also, it will stop the development of new cases.

Furthermore, we suggest to, in addition to the usage of remedies at home, avoid the use of caseums, take between one two and a half liters and 2 liters of water per daily, since saliva remains in continuous movement, it will be more difficult for develop bacteria in the mouth and throat area. of the throat and mouth.

Apply this wellness tip each time you have a caseum onto your tonsils in order to eliminate effortlessly and in a straightforward and natural manner.

Chapter 9: Tonsil Stones

Tonsil stones can also be referred to as tonsilloliths. They are extremely soft accumulations of cellular and bacterial matter that appears as tonsillar crypts as well as in the tonsil crevices. Tonsil stones typically occur within the tonsils of the palatine.

They can be present in the lingual tonsils. The condition is quite common and is affecting everyone irrespective the age. Tonsil stones have been reported as weighing of 0.3g up to 42g.

There are a variety of tonsil stones. All are a bit like unwanted objects that are stored within the tonsil crypt. Some times, tonsil stones can be an inconvenience and difficult to eliminate, but they're rarely dangerous. Tonsil stones can also be among the main causes for the halitosis condition or just bad breath. they are also a source stink that is pungent.

Tonsil stones are tough white or sometimes yellow-colored structures that are found in and around the tonsils. Most those who suffer from tonsil stones don't even aware of the existence of these stones. This is due to the fact that tonsil stones are usually not difficult to spot and can be found in a variety of sizes that range from rice-sized up to larger sizes of like large grapes.

It is important to note that tonsil stones are very rare and may cause more serious problems with health and cause complications. However it is possible that they develop into larger structures that can cause the tonsils to expand and produce a foul odor.

In contrast there are some cases where tonsil stones can cause discomfort and require them to be treated for tonsil stones. Tonsils are structures of the gland that are situated in the rear of the throat. Tonsils are inside a pocket of the throat along both sides.

Tonsils consist of tissues that contain lymphocytes, which are cells found in the body that help to fight diseases. Certain studies indicate that tonsils play an significant roles in human immunity and function as webs that are able to trap virus as well as bacteria passing through the throat.

Tonsil Stones Symptoms

In terms of signs of tonsil stones to be aware of, remember that in some cases, they don't cause signs at all. However it is possible that they are connected with bad breath, and other symptoms like the sensation of pain when taking a swallow.

While there might be none of the symptoms that could indicate that someone is suffering from tonsil stones CT scans or X-rays could quickly detect the presence of tonsil stones. However, tonsil stones that are huge by dimensions usually cause irritation to the throat, as well as bad breath.

One of the initial and most important indicators that indicate someone is suffering from tonsil stones is a unpleasant breath. This is also called Halitosis, which is usually a sign of tonsil infections. A study shows that with tonsil stones, odorless compounds typically happen.

It also revealed that a majority of the people with intense contractions of chemical compounds that smelled foul In reality, they were suffering from tonsil stones. The study also suggests that tonsil stones should be considered in every situation when there's no obvious motive for someone to develop smelly breath.

Another sign of tonsil stone is sore throat. When tonsil stones and tonsillitis also are present in the same period it can be difficult to identify what's the cause of sore throats, which is caused by the infection caused tonsil stones.

But, tonsil stones is often accompanied by irritation in the specific location where the stone has become in the throat, leading to sore throat.

Chapter 10: Causes Of Tonsil Stones

Concerning the factors that cause tonsil stones, the cause is blocking of substances like mucous and the cells that get trapped within tonsils. Tonsils are full of small nooks and crevices, and occasionally bacteria, along with various other materials, like dead cells can get caught.

If the situation occurs, this debris could easily be condensed in white tonsil formations in tonsil pockets. Tonsil stones can further form during the period when the the accumulation of debris hardens and calcifies.

It is more frequent in those suffering from some form of chronic inflammation that is located in their tonsils aswell in frequent episodes with tonsil stone. Note that the vast majority of patients have tonsil stones that are located within their tonsils.

In contrast individuals with tonsil stones and the type that is solidified seldom occur, however it likely. Tonsil stones are extremely common conditions that affect a huge variety of people, including adults and kids.

The primary reason that cause tonsil stones is due to the sulfur bacterias that easily get collected and the debris is trapped within the tonsils. The debris that is accumulated and stored comprise food particles, mucus as well as other substances.

The matter that decays accumulates and is stored into tiny crevices that are found in the tonils' surfaces. It is possible for this to cause the formation of multiple tonsils within the same region.

Tonsil Stones Treatment

If you are looking for methods to treat tonsil stones, you should know that most of them aren't dangerous, and in many instances treatment is not required. If patients have a lot of trouble with the smell of bad breath or sore throat that is brought on from tonsil stone, there's a variety of remedies that can alleviate discomfort and help in reducing bad breath.

Based on the level of severity for tonsil stone symptoms there are a variety of natural cures that are available and various treatments can be carried out by a doctor. One of the most popular medical treatments is the laser tonsil hydrolysis, a is a non-invasive treatment using lasers that gets rid of pockets and crevices that contain debris and substances trapped.

The procedure causes only a little sensation of. Local anesthesia can be used for ensuring patients receive a totally painless treatment. Oral irrigators can also be utilized to wash the crypts of tonsils. Another treatment option for treating medical conditions is Nimesulide that is used to treat tonsil stones. It is a mouthwash for oral use.

Natural Treatment of Tonsil Stones

There are also home remedies that are made from natural ingredients for relieving the sore throat and unpleasant breath that is due to tonsil stones. Apple cider vinegar, when mixed with water, can significantly ease the discomfort that are caused by tonsil stones. If you are suffering from tonsil stones it is advised to take probiotics.

A lemon juice drink is also a great option and can be extremely beneficial to eliminate tonsil stones. If you suffer from tonsil stones, it's a great idea to start eating organic, non-sweetened yogurt.

Drinks with a lot of fizz like soda could aid to eliminate tonsil stones as they break them down the same manner as apple cider breaks it. Apples, carrots, and onions can also be great home remedies that can aid in eliminating infections and help prevent oral infections as they have antibacterial qualities.

Chapter 11: What Are The Tonsil Stones?

Tonsil stone are calcifications that are formed in crypts that the

The palatal tonsils. Tonsil stones can also be found to develop inside the throat, and also in the roof in the mouth. Tonsils contain pockets where bacteria, as well as other material, like dead tissue.

mucus and cells, could get mucus and cells, can become trapped. While the role of the tonsils are not fully recognized, experts agree that they have an important immunity role in the child years.

Tonsils consist of lymphocytes, which are cells. When children are born, the lymphocytes create antibodies to help fight respiratory ailments. They shrink gradually by the time an individual attains puberty. However, they do not fully disappear completely. The position of the tonsils makes them able to snag on germs (viruses as well as bacteria). However, the immune function of the tonsils could be lost, their presence is a benefit.

In the absence of a cure for illness, adults, they may become more irritable due to the toxins and bacteria they accumulate. If this happens it can lead to tonsillitis. When it's severe and persistent it is possible to remove

Tonils (tonsillectomy) can be necessary. Although tonsil stones can appear to be a fake medical condition but they could cause serious problems. Tonsil stones are also known as tonsilliths and tonsilloliths

There are harmless accumulations of dirt and bacteria that can be found inside the crypts in some tonsils of people. However, this issue can lead to

It isn't hazardous and it is often treated.

How to Get Rid Of Tonsil Stones?

The correct treatment of an tonsil stone will depend on the

The size of the tonsillolith as well as the possibility of it causing discomfort or even medical damage. The options are numerous, including:

Treatment is not required. Numerous tonsil stones, particularly ones with symptoms and do not require any special treatment.

At-home removal. Some people choose to dislodge tonsil

Stones at home using the help of swabs or picks.

Salt water gargles. Gargling with warm salty water can ease the pain of tonsillitis which is often the result of

tonsil stones

Antibiotics. Different antibiotics are used for treating tonsil stones. While they might be useful to some, they are not recommended for everyone.

can't fix the root cause which causes tonsilloliths. In addition, antibiotics could cause adverse negative effects.

Removal surgically. If tonsil stones are extremely big and

If they are symptomatic, it might require surgery to get them removed. In some instances doctors will be capable of performing this procedure.

It is a relatively easy procedure that uses an numbing agent local to the area. After that, the patient with the tonsil stone won't require general anesthesia.

A good oral hygiene routine is the best way to protect yourself.

It is crucial in the prevention of these stones and also helping keep from developing nasty illnesses like gingivitis. Brushing

Also, flossing two every day, at a minimum is recommended. If feasible, brush and floss and rinse your mouth with your mouthwash at the end of every meal.

Oxygenating toothpaste eliminates bacteria.

Oxygenating toothpaste can be very beneficial for preventing tonsilloliths because it decreases the amount of bacteria present within the mouth.

Cleaning your tongue, gums and even the inside of your mouth

can eliminate all bacteria floating around.

Get your water flowing with water.

drinks that contain sugar may cause a film to form over the tonsils which could cause tonsil stones. Also, water can be active in removing

The yellow globs are prevented from forming mucus by washing away all food debris which you've eaten and is accumulating. It is a useful cost-effective, quick, and simple option.

Eat less food before bedtime.

Avoid eating if you plan to sleep within 30 minutes. Make sure you're cleaning your teeth thoroughly after eating the last meal or snack. In this way, you'll prevent any particles from entering your mouth.

of food items from colliding in your mouth when of you rest, which causes tonsiloliths.

Make sure you scrape your tongue.

In the course of one day Your tongue is a great place to collect food particles

bacteria as well as dead white blood cells and bacteria. A tongue scraper could assist to prevent tonsil stones since it removes

Eliminate all three reasons from your tongue as well as the mouth.

Gargle.

Gargling with a mouthwash helps in getting rid of any food particles that may have got stuck near the rear of your mouth.

throat. A mouthwash that is oxygenated helps in eliminating any bacteria that might exist. This could be like an effective two-in-one to prevent the formation of stones.

Garlic.

The chewing of garlic cloves is known to help remove stones naturally. The anti-bacterial properties of garlic can be used to aid in treating many ailments caused by bacteria, as well as tonsil stones.

are no different. You can chew on garlic a couple of every day. The garlic can help eliminate any bacterial matter that could be helping to solidify the substances in your tonsils.

Chapter 12: Lemon Juice

Lemon juice is a great source of vitamin C. It can assist in the removal of tonsil stones efficiently. What you have to mix is a couple of teaspoons of lemon juice into one cup of hot water. You can

"I removed tonsil stones from the comfort of my own home!"

My tonsil stones grew larger and bigger, and the odor was awful!

It was then that I came across an easy and painless method to disintegrate and eliminate my tonsil stone.

=This is what I came up with, make sure to check for yourself...

Add a small amount of salt in the lemon juice and make a drink.

Keep the juice of a lemon swirling over the areas affected by your tonsils prior to swallowing. Every time you drink, keep the lemon juice swirling around your tonsils.

Certain solutions suggest to keep it in your mouth for one time of at least a.

Fingers

If you're able to get your tonsils to your fingers, attempt to scrape your tonsils to remove the stones. Be careful, as picking at your stones in a way that is too vigorous could create more problems. If you do manage to scratch

Remove the stones and immediately start to gargle salt water in your mouth, to eliminate of any stones may have been loosening.

Essential Oils

Certain essential oils possess antibacterial and anti-inflammatory qualities that help with this problem. Certain of them

important oils that you ought to think about to use include myrrh, lemongrass and thieves oil.

Sprinkle a few drops the essential oil to your toothbrush every day

Every day, you should brush your tongue and teeth. There is also the option of purchasing the essential oils you need in spray bottles, and then apply the spray onto the area affected.

Yogurt

Eat unsweetened organic yogurt in order to eliminate the stones. Yogurt contains probiotics which are the healthy bacteria.

the body could require assist in the removal of tonsil stones to prevent them from returning. Yogurt that is natural and probiotic helps to eliminate microorganisms and other substances inside your tonsils.

that are responsible for the evolution for the development.

Apple Cider Vinegar

Any vinegar will assist in removing tonsil stones due to

vinegar contains acid. Acid will begin to devour the stones till they're completely broken. Utilize apple cider or white vinegar to aid you. Be sure to dilute the

Vinegar mixed with a tiny amount of water prior to when you start drinking.

Fizzy Beverages

Club soda and other fizzy drinks can be very beneficial for tonsil stone elimination because they dissolve the stones exactly like vinegar.

Apples

One of the most frequent causes for tonsil stones is bad oral hygiene. Because of the moderate acidic substance that apples have, these stones are

capable of acting as an astringent, and also help to clean your teeth. Additionally, when you chew them, they function as a brush, cleaning gums and your teeth and leaving them clear. Improve improve your oral health and rid of stones by eating apples.

Chapter 13: Carrots

Carrots are known to be beneficial for eyes thanks to the beta-carotene levels. In reality, chewing on carrots could assist in eliminating stone by eliminating the bacteria. The flow of saliva

The more you consume veggies like celery or carrots as this can help eliminate the bacteria that are in your mouth, which could cause the formation of stones.

Onions

Consuming raw onions can to improve the health of your mouth and help eliminate dental infections and bacteria since it's full of powerful anti-bacterial benefits. Make time to chew raw onions for 2 to three minutes every day and aid in removing and preventing tonsil stones. Additionally, onion chewing can assist remove the bad bacteria.

breath. It is often a manifestation of tonsil stone.

If tonsil stones cannot be manually taken out or resisted, they can cause serious problems.

breath may persist. It can become serious that one finds it difficult to communicate with relatives or friends. There are a variety of options to avoid this problem.

tonsil stones from developing and forming without the need to have your tonsils removed.

Tips for Reducing the Formation of Tonsil Stones

1. Make sure you clean your teeth and tongue at least twice per day

2. Cleanse your mouth using an oxygenating mouthwash

3. Take a drink after eating to flush the food particles which may be in the throat

4. Rinse the tonsils regularly by using an oral irrigator. This will keep bacteria and debris from building up in the crevices of your tonsils.

5. Clear nasal passages can reduce the incidence of postnasal drip.

The root cause behind tonsil stones

6. Avoid dairy-based products in your diet since they are high in protein which anaerobic bacteria thrives on.

7. Do not drink too much as alcohol is an

diuretic, which causes dry mouth.

Chapter 14: Do You Want To Eliminate Your Tonsil Stones?

Have you tried everything but nothing seems to have performed?

Read this tonsil stone guide to find out...

How can you rid yourself to tonsil stones?

What's the most effective way to rid yourself of tonsil stones?

Do tonsil stones disappear all on their own?

Are there any stones that can cause harm to you?

Are tonsil stone signs of cancer?

Are there tonsil stones that are normal?

How come people develop tonsil stone?

What can you do to prevent the formation of tonsil stone?

Are tonsil stones odorous?

Are tonsil stones either hard or soft?

Are there tonsil stones that are normal?

Are tonsil stones a sign that your breath is bad?

What is a tonsillolith?

Tonsils make up the part of our immune system that is responsible for that filter microorganisms such as viruses or bacteria, and harmful bacteria. If any is trying to infiltrate the body through the nose or mouth, the tonsils filter them out to stop their entrance.

In certain cases the contact with germs may cause the tonsils to get infected, and patients may be suffering from enflamed or inflamed tonsils. This is something called medically tonsillitis.

Tonsillitis is not to be confused with stone found in the tonsils. These are which are medically referred to as tonsilloliths, as well as the infections they trigger called tonsillitis.

Tonsilloliths occur due to calcium salts, or in combination with mineral salts which become trapped in the in the crypts (or craves) of the tonsils that are palatine. The crypts appear as small pockets that are visible on the surfaces of the tonsils being referred to as cryptic tonsils.

Coconut oil that is extra virgin is used for a long time not just for getting fresh breath but however, it can also help with additional oral issues, such as:

Stop bleeding gums.

Lower the risk of developing gum infection.

Smile with a white smile

Get healthy gums.

The growth of bacteria must be stopped inside the mouth.

There are several Internet videos that show huge pimples and pimples have been eliminated ... and well nowadays, the fashion is those videos that show stones within the tonsils.

The truth is that due to the enormous popularity of these films, many people are finding out for the first time, what are the stones inside the tonsils ... and the way they came to be.

If you're like so many others, have tonsils ... it's almost certain that at some point you'll have tonsils.

Without the wonders of YouTube without YouTube, I'd be unaware of their existence ... and perhaps I'd live a more tranquil life. The tonsils' stones or tonsilloliths can be the same just as the global climate change ... as well they're not nice in any way.

What exactly are they?

If you don't want to look at the videos, then don't bother doing it. It is as simple as this Think of a teratoma as an insidious twin which usually includes tiny teeth as well as hair, and may grow indefinitely without being noticed in the body for several years.

Think about the thing you've got within your mouth. If you are scared, those tonsil stones are not a teratoma however, they appear to be tiny tooth-like yellow teeth that are sticking out of the tonsils of your mouth, like you had a new collection of toothless teeth inside the throat.

Tonsilloliths consist of dead cells as well as mucous membranes that are trapped inside the tonsils. As time passes, they become hard and then turn yellowish.

"I Cured My Tonsil Stones in 3 Days"

I'm no longer required to swallow tonsil stones, sore throats or the unpleasant dragon breath. It was done with the most basic natural cure.

==> Here Is What I Did...

If the photo of these stones fails to make you feel like you are in the waves ... take a look that the stones within these stones aren't simply stones. They're part of a bacterial carpet (biofilm).

If you're reading this, it's true that your stones are living! What's more is unlike an teratoma don't have hair.

What can I do to tell if are suffering from stones?

Easy. The first thing you'll notice is unpleasant breath. You may also experience signs like the sore throat, white or whitish residues and difficulty swallowing. You may also experience irritation in the ears, and tonsil inflammation.

What can I do to get off my shoes?

Though they tend to are able to fall off on their own but you could also try taking them off yourself like you can in the video, or gargle them with salt water. If this doesn't work then they will need be surgically removed (and perhaps record the procedure to upload it on YouTube).

If you suspect you may are suffering from tonsilloliths but don't want to stick your

hands on it or even consult an expert,
I've got bad news for ya The bad stink
will not go away.

Chapter 15: The Signs Of Stone Within The Tonsils

There are several various indicators that can indicate that someone is suffering from tonsil stones, which could include these:

A metallic taste is present in the mouth

Halitosis that is recurrently present, and associated with a throat infection

The cough can be a source of discomfort.

Then close or tighten the throat

Suffocation

It is difficult to swallow

The throat is swollen

Causes

There is no explanation for why they occur They are also uncommon. Some of the motives for why they appear include:

Dental hygiene and hygiene of the mouth are rather bad

The residues from the actions of enzymes present in stored foods. They can create an accumulation of bacteria on the food particles which then get stored in the crypts the tonsils in the palatine.

Oral bacteria

The salivary glands are hyperfunctioning.

Mucus secretion is a part of the mucus production process.

Leukocytes (white blood cells) dead.

Smoking with no filter

Eliminate tonsil crystals and bad breath due to food particles

Most importantly, tonsilloliths generally are nothing more than sound. They are sometimes removed when they're removed from their tonsils. If you're fortunate, there are alternative options.

"I Cured My Tonsil Stones in 3 Days"

It's no longer necessary to cough up tonsil stone, sore throats or a nasty breath of dragon. It was done with an easy remedy that is natural.

==> Here Is What I Did...

If you're still not fortunate, you can try other ways to get lucky.

It isn't easy to remove them however it is possible to get accomplished. Try the job by extricating them using your brush or fingers (ouch!) A different option is using the Q-tip. The final option is to clean using the water comb. It can be described as a pressure irrigator that is used in dentistry.

The water comb may be utilized to remove food that is stuck in the tonsils. The particles clean food particles out between teeth. The theory is that it performs better than flossing. You can also use special sprays and nasal drops that you are able to use to stop these.

Treatment for tonsillitis with a medical doctor

If someone is suffering from fevers or difficulties swallowing, it's important to seek medical assistance. There is a possibility that there is a need for antibiotics or anti-inflammatory medications.

It's usually a 10-day regimen of antibiotics in order in order to treat the disease.

In the most extreme instances, if it becomes impossible for an individual to swallow food because the tonsils have swelled and there are stones inside the tonsils, they can be admitted to hospital and given intravenous fluids.

Surgery to remove the tonsils: This procedure occurs when someone was treated with tonsils for stones but and had no results over the course of the course of a year, or when they show the most severe signs.

Tonsilloliths tend to be more prevalent when patients suffer of chronic tonsillitis. When this happens surgeries or tonsillectomy are considered as final option, since taking out the tonsils is similar to the elimination of a portion of the immune system.

The physician will administer a local anesthetic and will then remove the tonsils via surgical procedure. The procedure can provide permanent relief to someone who's suffered from swelling of the tonsils and stones for quite a while.

DRINK A LOT OF WATER

If you drink enough water, your body is hydrated making it more difficult for bacteria to live. A regular intake of water on an ongoing routine will help remove the tonsils, and stop their accumulation and the formation of stone in them.

Chapter 16: Wear A Cotton Hisopo

You can also utilize cotton swabs. Make sure to moisten the edges of the cotton swabs take a flashlight and place it before an mirror.

Utilize the swabs to gently move the stones around and take them away from your tonsils.

Then, rinse with mouthwash or saltwater to eliminate any the particles and debris.

Tonsil stones are comprised of all the debris that is accumulated within the tonsils. The tonsils are glands behind the throat. They have tonsillar crypts, or folds.

Calcium and other minerals and mucus and dead cells may build up in these folds, and form small, white spots. The fungi and bacteria which affect the tonsils and trigger tonsillitis can contribute to the formation of these stones.

Garlic

It is well-known that garlic offers many advantages for medical care. You can simply chew garlic and remove stones without difficulty and efficiently.

It is recommended to chew garlic at least once a throughout the day. It also helps to fight off bacteria that may aid in the formation of the substances in the tonsils.

Lemon juice

Lemon juice is among the most natural cures for tonsil stones. Lemon juice has a lot of vitamin C which helps to in the removal of tonsil stones.

For the use of lemon juice in the treatment for tonsil stone, mix a few tablespoons of lemon juice into hot water in a cup. Add a bit of salt into the lemon juice as well as drinks.

www.ingramcontent.com/pod-product-compliance
Lightning Source LLC
Chambersburg PA
CBHW060243030426
42335CB00014B/1585